Crib Sheets
New Parent Sleep Solutions
Practical and Effective Strategies

Elizabeth Gardner

Copyright 2002, 2003, 2009, 2021 by Elizabeth Gardner

THIS BOOK WAS PREVIOUSLY PUBLISHED AS "Crib Sheets® Are You Covered? New Parent Sleep Deprivation Solutions: Practical and Effective Expectant Parent Strategies

Fourth Edition

ISBN-13: 9798718427523

No portion of this book may be reproduced in any form without permission from the author, except as permitted by U.S. copyright law. Every effort has been made by the author and publishing house to ensure that the information contained in this book was correct as of press time. The author and publisher hereby disclaim and do not assume liability for any injury, loss, damage, or disruption caused by errors or omissions, regardless of whether errors or omissions result from negligence, accident, or any other cause. Readers are encouraged to verify any information contained in this book prior to taking any action on the information.
For rights and permissions, please contact:
Elizabeth Gardner neonpinklime@gmail.com

Contents

Chapter One: Maximize Your Sleep With Baby 1

Chapter Two: Adults Are On Their Own 8

Chapter Three: Siblings Are Self-Reliant 16

Chapter Four: Reduce Time Spent On Bills And Appointments .. 25

Chapter Five: Keep Car Trips To A Minimum 31

Chapter Six: Quick And Easy Family Travel 40

Chapter Seven: Fast And Frustration Free Cooking With Baby ... 48

Chapter Eight: Duplicate Useful Tools And Locate Strategically 59

Chapter Nine: What Next? 65

Chapter Ten: Sleepless Nights With Baby 66

Chapter Eleven: The Won't Stop Crying Baby 68

About the Author 70

Chapter One

MAXIMIZE YOUR SLEEP WITH BABY

1. Do tasks that can be done with baby awake only when baby is awake.

2. Reduce tasks that must be done with baby asleep in number and duration.

3. Purchase baby items to safely bring baby along while doing household tasks.

4. Set up items to help bring baby along where daily household tasks are performed.

1. Do tasks that can be done with baby awake only when baby is awake.

The truth is that caring for a newborn will be one of the most difficult things you will ever do. Most new moms have various aches and pains to deal with post-delivery including hemorrhoids, episiotomy or C-section stitches, and bleeding. There's also the steep learning curve that comes with a new baby; for example, difficulty and pain breastfeeding can cause anxiety and frustration. Changing hormone levels are another adjustment for new moms. Fluctuating hormones can cause mood swings that result in depression, and, of course, there's the newborn to adjust to as well. Their relentless and persistent cries can cause anxiety and feelings of failure and frustration for both mom and dad. But it's the constant mind-numbing fatigue caused by two-hour feedings that makes dealing with these circumstances so very hard. In the midst of it all parents think to themselves, "Maybe I could handle this if only I could get more sleep?"

In the before time, sleep was simple: when you felt tired, you went to bed. Once baby arrives, however, deciding when and how long to sleep are no longer your decisions—or at least not yours alone. Baby's feedings and temperament control when and for how long parents sleep, and for the first few months, newborns sleep unpredictably and for short intervals. Your newborn will feed 8 to 12 times a day or, in other words, every two to three hours.[1] And although feeding times gradually stretch to every three to four hours after one month of age, exactly when that happens varies from infant to infant.[2] That means at least one parent will suffer months of serious sleep deprivation. Even if you decide to bottle feed, one parent, or both if you take turns, will be feeding and burping baby every two to three hours, twenty-four hours a day. It's exhausting.

---

[1] See, US Department of Health and Human Services office on Woman's Health Web site at http://womanshealth.gov/breastfeeding.

[2] Ibid.

What can parents do to get more sleep? Most baby experts focus on ways to make baby somehow sleep longer. They suggest keeping the home quiet, darkening baby's room, or avoiding diaper changes if she wakes to feed. Although this advice may help baby fall asleep, it is unlikely to make a baby sleep longer because newborns eat every two hours. Experts also suggest that tired parents forego household chores. Let the dishes and laundry pile up and sleep instead they say. Realistically, however, parents can't do that for very long. Grocery shopping, cooking, and bill paying are just a few of the many tasks that cannot be postponed. I agree with baby experts as far as they go—yes, if you're tired and have the opportunity to sleep then don't do household chores. But this advice goes only so far. The fact is that someone has to shop, make meals, and pay the bills. Even if you and your spouse split work and household responsibilities fifty-fifty, they still need to get done.

So, how can parents get more sleep? By making decisions based on their own actions rather than those of an uncontrollable newborn. Since baby sleep time is parent free or sleep time, you want to protect that time while also taking maximum advantage of it. That means reducing and eliminating tasks that must be done while baby sleeps and doing them only when baby is awake. Once you've done all you can to eliminate and reduce tasks that must be done while baby sleeps, you'll only get the most sleep possible if you stop performing tasks while baby sleeps that can be done with baby awake.

This is a sensible and well-balanced approach to tackling the problem of parent sleep deprivation; namely, focus on controlling your own actions as parents rather than the actions of an uncontrollable newborn. If you accept the fact that your baby is going to do whatever they want and you organize your tasks and free time accordingly, you'll be a lot more productive, a lot less frustrated, and get more sleep. The best time to prepare is before baby arrives when you'll have both time and energy to prepare; however, once baby arrives, it's not too late. You can still implement *Crib Sheets'* sleep maximization techniques to get the most sleep possible. If you already have a newborn, for example, not wasting baby sleep time doing tasks that can be done with baby along will immediately get you more sleep

At this moment, I'm sitting here writing this book. I have a three-month-old daughter who's asleep. I also have a sink full of dirty dishes, a full dishwasher in need of unloading, dirty laundry waiting in the laundry room, clean laundry in my washing machine, dry laundry in my dryer, and the downstairs needs vacuuming. Why am I not tending to these tasks? *Because they are things I can do while baby is awake.* If you see a chore that needs to be done, ask yourself if it can wait until baby is awake. If so, don't do it if baby is asleep. This takes some discipline. I don't know how many times I've started to wash dishes and remembered, "The baby is asleep!" I've had to stop myself mid-chore and redirect my energy toward my personal interests. Baby sleep time is your time. Protect it. Don't waste it doing things that you and your baby can do together. I use my time when baby sleeps to catch up on my own sleep, write, or read. These are things that I want to do and enjoy doing but absolutely cannot do with baby awake.

2. Reduce tasks that must be done with baby asleep in number and duration.

How do you decide whether a household task can be performed with baby awake? By determining whether or not it requires more than 15 minutes of uninterrupted concentration. Once fed and changed, most babies stay content for about 15 minutes. I call this the "baby contentment window." If a household chore requires more than 15 minutes of uninterrupted concentration, and is therefore beyond the baby contentment window, it either cannot be done with baby awake or would be much easier to do with baby asleep. For instance, paying bills, phone calls to creditors, writing a grocery list, grocery shopping, meal preparation, and clothes shopping are activities requiring longer periods of concentration. A few of them such as writing a grocery list, grocery shopping, and meal preparation can be interrupted to soothe baby but doing so repeatedly makes completion difficult. Since these tasks are much easier when

> *If a task requires more than 15 minutes of uninterrupted concentration, then it is much easier to do with baby asleep. Prepare now to minimize such tasks both in number and duration.*

baby sleeps, performing them takes away parent sleep or free time; therefore, you want to spend as little time and effort as possible on these tasks. Chapter Four "Minimize Bill Payment and Appointment and Time," and Chapter Five "Keep Car Trips to a Minimum" explain how.

Once you maximize free time by doing only the chores you must while baby sleeps and doing them in the least amount of time possible, you can extend your free time even further by minimizing or eliminating interruptions. You'll be able to sleep longer with fewer interruptions, for example, if adults and children in your household are self-reliant. Self-reliance saves time because when others do for themselves, then less needs to be done. Adult and child self-reliance are the focus of Chapter Two "Adults are on their Own" and Chapter Three "Siblings are Self-Reliant."

What about tasks that take only 15 minutes or, if longer, can be interrupted to soothe baby? Do these with baby. This chapter as well as Chapter Six "Quick and Easy Family Travel," Chapter Seven "Fast and Frustration Free Cooking with Baby," and Chapter Eight "Duplicate Useful Tools and Locate Strategically" will help you bring baby along and suggest ways to make such tasks easier.

3. Buy baby items to safely bring baby along while doing household chores.

Many tasks can be performed that are within the 15-minute "baby contentment window" like filling or emptying the dishwasher, clothes washing or folding or putting away, or making a bed. Take baby with you for these. For chores that take longer than 15 minutes and interrupting to soothe baby

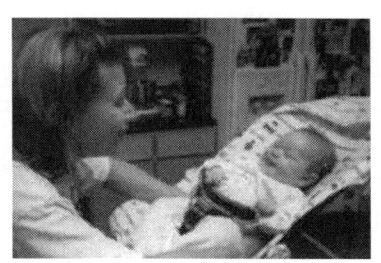

Baby bouncer seat in kitchen vibrates to soothe while doing dishes and other chores.

doesn't make completion too difficult, for example, vacuuming, dusting, or cleaning a bathroom, also bring baby along. Tasks like vacuuming and dusting, for instance, don't take a lot of thought. Once the interruption is over, it's easy to simply pick up where you left off. Since they are basically mindless tasks, they are perfect to do with baby along, and doing them only with baby awake maximizes your sleep time.

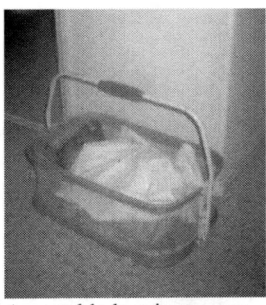

There are baby products that make doing housework with baby easier. These products provide a safe place to put baby, freeing your hands for other tasks. Baby bouncer seats, for example, are safe for baby and can be carried from chore to chore. You can even purchase ones that vibrate or make music to soothe. Similarly, a Moses basket, portable bassinet, or infant swing can provide a temporary spot for baby. These items work well in areas of the home without carpet or where there's no safe or clean place to put baby. Playmats and gyms are great for carpeted areas where baby is able to lie safely such as bedroom, dining rooms, and living rooms. Front packs work well anywhere but especially when tasks require a lot of movement from room to room, for instance, vacuuming, dusting, or cooking.

A portable bassinette can be carried from task to task.

Doing housework with baby provides an opportunity for the two of you to interact. Take advantage of it. Smile and talk to baby while you work. Tell baby about all the laundry you're doing or the dishes you're washing. If baby starts to fuss, stop doing laundry or dishes, or whatever, and soothe them. Once they quiet down, resume your work. If they fall asleep, then stop doing your work and enjoy your free time by sleeping or doing something fun. Resume the task when baby wakes.

> *To save money, consider buying baby items second hand at garage sales, swap meets, online, or via classified ads. For instructions, print them from the Web.*

4. Set up items to help bring baby along where daily household tasks are performed.

Identify where most of your daily chores are performed and set up devices allowing you to bring baby along. In my home, most of the daily chores are performed in the laundry room and kitchen. I have a vibrating bouncer seat in my kitchen for baby when I'm cooking or cleaning up. When I need to do laundry, I carry the bouncer seat into the laundry room, or I lay baby down on a playmat on the carpeted floor in the hallway within sight of the washer and dryer.

Determine what baby devices you can safely put in your housework areas. If there's carpet, then perhaps a playmat or gym is a good idea. Try a bouncer seat, portable bassinet or infant swing if there's no carpet. If you want to vacuum with baby, then a front or backpack may be best. Buy and set up now so you'll be ready whenever baby arrives. If baby is already here, then strategically place your devices to get chores done with your little one in tow.

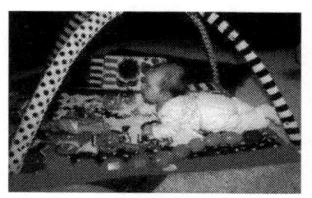

Playmat works well on carpet.

Chapter Two

ADULTS ARE ON THEIR OWN

1. Deal with your own relatives.

2. See to household needs spontaneously.

3. Say "no" to adults outside the home.

4. Maintain your own vehicle, for example, oil change, or car repair.

5. Take care of your own plants and pets.

6. Make your own breakfast, lunch, and clean it up.

7. Do your own laundry, all or part, including folding, putting away, ironing, and dry cleaning.

My husband Paul and I ushered our two young sons down the aisle of a packed 727. We'd been looking forward to this Cape Cod vacation for months; now we sought sanity. A flight attendant's voice chattered over the intercom, "Ladies and gentlemen, if you would please clear the aisle and find your seats, we could depart." I buckled Eiche ("Ike") and Max in between us. Paul searched their backpack for something to keep them busy. A flight attendant demonstrated an oxygen mask, "Assist yourself so that you can better assist your child." I opened a pack of gum. "Can I have some?" Paul asked. I smiled and popped some into my mouth. "Assist yourself so that you can better assist your husband," I teased.

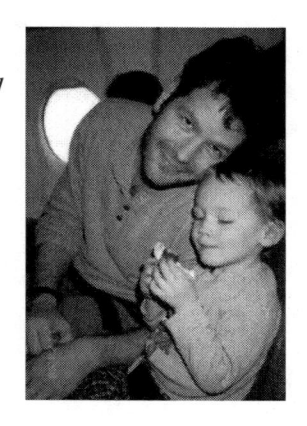

A happy parent is a better parent, so it's essential to make your happiness top priority. That means time for yourself to sleep, read, eat, paint, build, surf, or whatever. As a caregiver in your home, you may find this difficult. Undoubtedly, you're used to thinking of the needs of others before your own. But let's put this in perspective: how can you be happy and stay that way if you keep ignoring your needs? Having a baby is a miraculous experience, but it's a part of your life—not your whole life. You became a parent to enhance your life not replace it. When a new baby arrives, my top priorities are time to mother, sleep, and write. My baby is here, and I have the time I need. How? Because I discovered ways to cultivate enough free time to get the sleep I need and do the things I love. You can too!

A good way to create more time for yourself is to insist that adults in your home do things for themselves. Now, I'm not talking about chores that you and your spouse allocate between you. If you agreed on a household division of labor or decided that one spouse will do more chores than the other until baby is older that's great, but it's not what I mean. I'm talking about taking responsibility for your own needs with the reasonable expectation that other adults will do the same. For example, it's common for the primary childcare giver, usually mom, to assume some of the personal responsibilities of their spouse or other capable adults within the home such as making breakfast or lunch, folding or putting away laundry, making appointments, taking clothes to the dry cleaners, refilling the toilet paper dispenser, and so on. If this is true in your home, then it's time to give those responsibilities to whom they belong. A new baby means that adults are on their own.

Don't exempt relatives who stay in your home to share in the birth. They're capable adults, so treat them as such. Make it clear that they're not "guests" to be "entertained," but family who can see to their own needs as much as possible by doing their own laundry, making a meal, or cleaning their bathroom. Ask them to make dinner or babysit. If they're unwilling to at least take care of themselves during this physically and emotionally draining time, then perhaps a day visit is in order and not an extended stay. To save time and emotional upset, don't forget to let your spouse deal with their relatives while you deal with yours. (See number 1 below.)

> It can be difficult to let adults do things for themselves, especially when they struggle, but remember they are capable of fulfilling their own needs. Let them.

As is often the case, easier said than done. It's easy to tell other adults within the home that they must do for themselves; the hard part is going to be for you to let them. Watching them flounder is difficult, but you have to let them. If you ask them to do things for themselves while you continue doing for them, then they won't be self-reliant, and you'll be run ragged. If your wife forgets to water her plants, then let them die. If your husband forgets to get his laundry, then let it pile up. If you've shown your in-laws where the food, dishes, and utensils are but they refuse to fix themselves something to eat, then let them go hungry. These people are capable of fulfilling their own needs—let them.

What the primary caregiver doesn't do around the house will determine what other adults do for themselves. As the "doer" in your home, the decision rests in your hands because you have the power to stop doing. Think this over in terms of what's fair to you and others. Hold a house meeting to discuss what things you want to stop doing and why. In my home, I do things for my husband that can be done quickly and easily as part of what I do for the rest of the family. Simply put, if a task for my husband cannot be quickly and easily incorporated into my responsibilities regarding daily care of the kids, then I don't do it. I don't know all the things my husband does for himself because he does whatever he can for himself by himself. I'm not involved. What a relief!

1. Deal with your own relatives.

Let your spouse handle disagreements with their own parents, and you handle yours. This prevents misunderstandings and arguments requiring time and effort to repair. I'm talking about avoiding family feuds. Parents love their children no matter what, so no matter what you say to your parents they'll still love you. This isn't true for your in-laws. Emotionally charged issues like holiday plans, money, or adult sibling problems are best left for each spouse to discuss with their parents or relatives. Limit your contact with your spouse's parents or other relatives to pleasant conversations and babysitting arrangements.

Consider my friend Tonya's dilemma. She felt so huge and tired that she couldn't wait for baby to arrive. She also couldn't wait for her in-laws to leave. They came to live-in a week before her due date in order to "help out." They did help in some respects; for example, they picked up her older daughter from school. The problem was that they expected to be waited on and cleaned up after. Even though Tonya showed them where the dishes and food were, they refused to make themselves a

If relatives are unwilling to take care of themselves when they come to share in the birth, then maybe a day visit is in order; not an overnight stay.

meal. She would make a meal for herself, sit down to eat it, and they would sit at the table with her commenting how good it smelled. She would remind them again to "help themselves," but they would only sit there uncomfortably, so she'd stop eating, make some for them, and then clean it up. Of course, I thought this was nuts. I asked, "What do you think is going to happen after the baby is born?" She replied, "That's what I'm worried about." She also told me that they would neither clean their own bathroom nor do their own laundry, even though she asked them to. She wanted her husband to speak to them about the situation, but he'd always had trouble talking to them, and this time was no exception.

This illustrates a difficult problem: a spouse who won't deal with their own relatives. But just because they won't doesn't absolve them of the responsibility. It's their burden; *don't take it on.* As discussed earlier, you're not their child, therefore, if you approach your in-laws with issues it will result in turmoil that's difficult and time consuming to repair. Remember, no matter what your spouse says to them, they will still love them, not you.

Tonya needed to do two things. First, concentrate on doing what was within her power. Namely, stop cooking for them, stop cleaning up after them, and stop feeling guilty about it. They would start doing for themselves, her husband would do it, or it wouldn't get done. In any event, it would put the responsibility where it belongs. Second, she needed to explain to her husband that it was unfair to her for his parents to live-in if he's unable to deal with them. Maybe it would be best for them to stay in a hotel when they visit? Fine. His parents are his responsibility; let him handle them.

2. See to household needs spontaneously.

When I was eight months pregnant with my third child, I was sitting at the kitchen table eating dinner when Paul got up to throw something away. The trash was full, so he balanced it on top. It slid this way and that, but once the item was successfully "balanced" he walked away. I practically leapt out of my chair. "You cannot be serious!" Paul smiled a sort of "you caught me" smile and, without a word, removed the full bag and replaced it.

This is what I'm talking about when I suggest that adults should meet household needs without prompting. I'm talking about spontaneously doing all the little things around the home that everyone ignores, and the primary caregiver ends up doing. Let's be honest. Isn't this going on in your home? Adults are throwing trash into full trash receptacles, leaving toilet paper and paper towel rollers

> *Explain to adult family members that if they discover something in the home that needs attention, e.g., full trash basket, empty toilet paper roller, etc., that you expect them to give it their attention.*

empty, waiting for someone else to change the bathroom towels, not watering the plants or feeding the dog, and so forth. With a new baby there's neither time nor energy for these shenanigans. This has to stop, but how?

It's simple. Tell them, "Turn on your radar for tasks that need doing." Explain that if you find yourself using something that requires attention, then you expect them to give it their attention. If you use the last sheet of toilet paper, for example, then replace it, or if you use the last paper towel, put a new roll out, or if the trash is full, then replace it with a new bag. There are so many small household tasks requiring attention that it's impossible to list them all. That's why capable family members need to put this into practice now pre-baby so that you'll have more time and energy after. Meet with the adults in your household and explain why and how they must do more.

3. Say "No" to adults outside the home.

With the demands of a new baby, your time will be more limited and precious than ever. Learn to say "no" firmly and politely to outside requests. "No" is such an important word because it safeguards your time and sanity. Say it as often as you need to protect yourself. Emotionally healthy individuals will not dislike you simply because you say "no" so start saying it and clear your schedule before and after baby arrives.

> *Emotionally healthy individuals will not dislike you simply because you say "no," so start saying it and clear your schedule before baby arrives.*

Invitations to coach kids' sports, volunteer in the community, run or stock a snack bar, engage in a lengthy phone conversation, or have a long chat with neighbors can be great fun but are almost certainly too time consuming given a new baby. I enjoy volunteering in my kindergartner's classroom, but I stopped two months before my daughter was born. I miss it, so I'll be volunteering again when she's about six months. If outside commitments are important to you, remember that you'll have more time to give when your baby is sleeping longer and more regularly. But for now, evaluate each request in terms of whether it's important enough to take on. In the majority of situations, I've found that what people want me to do is either something I'm not interested in or, if interested, something which is not important enough to do when I'm sleep deprived from baby care.

Don't forget to say "no" to extended family outside the home as well. There will be relatives who cannot come see the baby but want you to drive or fly to see them. Since adjusting to your new family member is exhausting, a long-distance trip shortly after baby's birth may not be the best idea, or perhaps extended family want you to host a holiday dinner or undertake some other large family obligation after baby is born. Say "no" to your relatives. Your spouse can say "no" to theirs.

4. Maintain your own vehicle, for example, oil change or car repair.

Let adults take care of their own cars.

5. Take care of your own plants and pets.

If plants and pets in your home were adopted by both of you, then you should rightly share in the responsibility. But if another adult brings plants and/or pets into the home, then let them take care of them. Early in our marriage, Paul adopted a cat which he cared for. During the years before the kids came, I gradually took over cleaning the litter box and feeding, but once I was pregnant with our first child Paul reclaimed the responsibility. Our plant situation is similar. Paul loves plants, and he has lots of them. He takes care of them. Sometimes he forgets and ends up with dead plants. It's a matter of deciding what's important and making choices. Plants are not important to me; therefore, I don't buy them. Taking care of plants would take time away from doing things I care about.

6. Make your own breakfast, lunch, and clean it up.

Preparing breakfast and lunch for the family typically requires individual meals made separately, for instance, sandwiches, cereal, and toast. It can take even more time if adults and kids don't want the same sandwich or cereal or whatever. In contrast, dinner is traditionally a shared meal consisting of a single main course, for example, spaghetti, pot roast, or baked chicken. In other words, when it comes to dinner, the preparer usually doesn't have to make individual meals. Since it takes a lot of time to make each person breakfast and lunch, my husband makes his own. When he's done, I don't clean up his mess. He does. For ways to shorten meal prep time, please see Chapter Seven "Fast and Frustration Free Cooking with Baby"

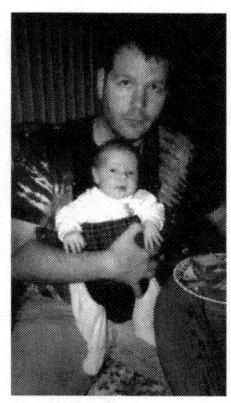

Paul totes baby Lauren in a front pack while making and eating lunch.

7. Do your own laundry including folding, putting away, ironing, and dry cleaning.

Let your spouse take responsibility for their clothes. In my home, I wash everyone's dirty laundry because it can be done in bulk in the washing machine. It doesn't require very much extra time to simply include my husband's clothes in the wash. But folding and putting away are another story. Paul folds his own clothes and puts them away. When he runs out, then he knows to go to the laundry room, fold his clothes, and put them away.

Avoid buying clothes that require ironing or dry cleaning. They waste too much time. If your spouse buys clothes requiring ironing or dry cleaning, then they can do it themselves.

Chapter Three

SIBLINGS ARE SELF-RELIANT

1. Children help each other.

2. Children two-and-a-half to three-years-old are toilet trained.

3. Children two-and-a-half-years-old dress and undress themselves including jacket and shoes.

4. Children two-and-a half-years-old get themselves a cup of water.

5. Children three-years-old throw out their trash in the house or car.

6. Children three-years-old wash and dry their hands.

7. Children three-years-old prepare a simple snack for themselves like as an apple or banana.

8. Children three-years-old use the TV remote on/off and tune in favorite channels.

9. Children four-years-old put dirty dishes by the sink.

10. Children two-and-a-half-years-old play in a single room and clean up their toys

A new baby means exhaustion. Small tasks easily dealt with pre-baby are now major interruptions when getting baby to sleep or catching up on your own, so the more big brother or sister can do for themselves, the better. Self-reliance brings pride and self-esteem to them and extra time to you.

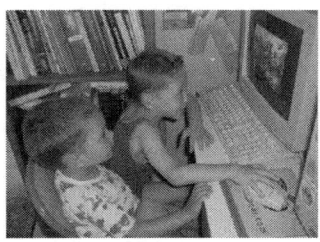

The list at the beginning of this chapter suggests ages at which children can master certain skills. My kids were capable of mastering these skills at those ages, so it's reasonable to assume yours can too. Even if you think your kids aren't ready, give them the opportunity to try. Children can surprise you.

Big brother Eiche (age five) helps Max (age three) on his computer.

1. Children help each other.

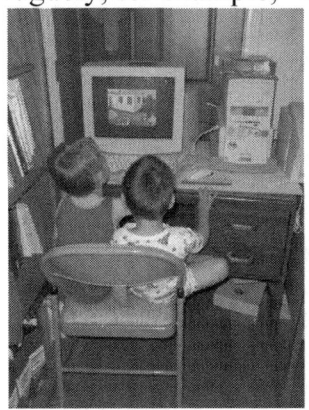

One of the best things about being in a family is that members help each other. Usually, parents communicate this to children vaguely, for example, "Go help your brother." Be more explicit. Explain to your kids that family members help one another. Tell them that when their brother or sister has trouble, they are expected to help. Certainly, kids feel great pride when they pitch in, but there are benefits beyond such as children learn to give and receive help as a way of life; kids become comfortable asking for help as well as offering it; family members learn they can trust each other; in other words, if they ask for help then they will receive it, and parents don't have to fix every child's problem themselves. This benefits the family not only now when troubles are small, for example, Trudy ran out of toilet paper, but also when your kids are adults and their troubles are somewhat larger. Family members learn that they can count on each other now and in the future.

Children helping each other helps you in any situation in which you cannot or would much rather not stop what you're doing, for example, soothing baby, rocking to sleep, changing diaper, or bathing baby. Kids can help each other get dressed, find toys, play on the computer, go to the bathroom, get a drink of water, clean up toys, color, throw things away, and so on. Eventually, your kids will start solving problems without you—just what you want if you've been up all night caring for baby.

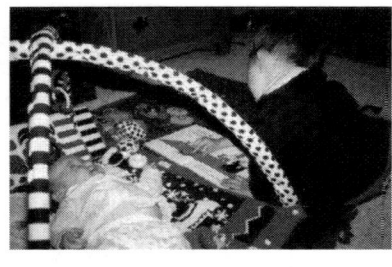

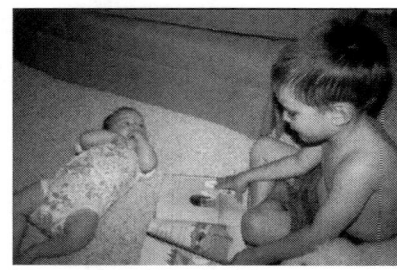

Max reads to little sister Lauren at two mos. and again at three mos.

2. Children two-and-a-half to three-years-old are toilet trained.

There is no denying that toilet training means one extremely important thing—freedom from the time, expense, and mess of diapers. Toilet training takes a few weeks to accomplish, so try a few months before baby arrives. A toddler that uses a toilet saves parents so much time that you should make the attempt to teach them even if you aren't sure they're ready. At two and a half, Eiche told me he had to "wee" while in the shower, so I told him to wee in the drain. He did. This demonstrated

Consider skipping the potty seat and training directly on the toilet. Put a lightweight stool in the bathroom, so toddler can use it to climb onto the toilet. It's easier to simply flush the waste away than it is to clean a potty seat. Plus, if they learn on the toilet, then you won't have to transition them from a potty chair, and when you're out, your child can use any toilet (without potty seat).

anticipation and control, so I thought he was ready to toilet train. He was. I toilet trained my other two kids at two and a half as well.

3. Children two-and-a-half-years-old dress and undress themselves including jacket and shoes.

If you've been dressing and undressing your two-and-a-half-year-old (or older) child, why not stop and let her try? Don't forget to praise what a big girl she is, and, if you can live with some odd color combinations, why not let her select her own clothes? Be sure to show your kids that clothes go in the hamper or laundry room when they're done wearing them.

Let's discuss shoes. I can't imagine why any parent would want to service their child's feet all day but some do. Just the other day, my five-year-old son had a friend over to play. Before they began, the kids took their shoes off. A half hour later, we decided to go out for lunch. My son put his sneakers on and tied his laces. My son's friend came to me to put his shoes on. I told him to put them on his feet, and I would tie the laces. He told me he couldn't. I tried and even I had difficulty simply getting them on his feet! It wasn't that the shoes were

> *An easy way to help a child learn to put on a jacket: put the hood of the jacket on first. This centers the jacket, lining it up for their arms. They then reach back and insert their arms into the sleeves.*

> *Help kids tell the right shoe from the left by showing them that Velcro closes toward the outside of the foot.*

too small for him; it was that they were just hard to get on. Once I got them on, then I tied laces too. We ate out, came back, and they removed their shoes to play. A short time later, they wanted to play outside. This meant shoes back on. Once again, I had to help our guest get shoes on and tied. Back inside a short time later, and the kids took their shoes off. Then they wanted to go out again. I put his friend's shoes on again. Back inside for the final hour, and they removed their shoes. When it was time to bring our young guest home, I had to put his shoes on and tie laces yet again, and I thought to myself: "For Pete's sake, how can your parents stand servicing your feet all day?"

A five-year-old that hasn't learned to tie laces yet is understandable, but at least they should be able to get shoes on their feet. When you take kids shoe shopping, make sure they can get the shoes on and off by themselves before you buy them. If your child hasn't learned to tie laces yet, and you're not ready to teach them, then buy shoes that close with Velcro or zipper, so you don't have to tie and re-tie laces.

> *Kids grow quickly. Keep a box in the child's closet for "outgrown clothes." Store it, give it to charity, or pass it down to a sibling or other relative*

Tying laces is a skill all kids eventually master. I've found that mine had the coordination at about five years of age. Give your kids the opportunity to practice. One of my kids learned to tie their sneakers after a kindergarten homework assignment required them to tie their laces twenty times in a row.

4. Children two-and-a-half-years-old can get themselves a cup of water.

When Eiche was two and a half, I accompanied him on a toddler school outing to a local park. At snack time the teachers handed out paper cups for juice. Eiche was accustomed to sippy cups, so he didn't know how to use it. That day, I held the cup up for him whenever he wanted a drink. Upon hearing me complain that I should have brought a sippy cup, an older, more experienced mom walked up beside me and said, "You know when our moms raised us, they didn't have these no spill sippy cups they have today." I told her, "I would transition him to a cup, but I'm dreading the spills he'll make all over the house." She replied, "What our moms used to do was confine eating and drinking to the kitchen table. If a kid wanted a drink that's where they would drink it, not carry it around with them." What a sensible idea! In order to minimize mess, not only should eating be a kitchen table activity but drinking as well. I went home, threw out my sippy cups, and told my kids that all eating and drinking would be done at the kitchen table. Then I

> *A refrigerator with a built-in exterior water dispenser makes it easier for kids to get themselves a cup of water.*

taught them how to drink from a cup. Sure, we had some spills but less and less over time. When there were spills, they were confined to the kitchen.

If you have one or more kids that use a "sippy cup," that's a cup with a special screw or pop on no spill top, consider weaning to a regular cup. Although it may seem easier to let them use a sippy cup because it can be carried without spills, consider the big downside—they can't get their own drink. If you teach them to use a regular cup, then almost any available cup will work at home or when eating out. Additionally, drinking from a cup is a skill they must learn at some point, so why not before baby arrives? If your child asks for juice, it's easier to say, "I can't get juice right now but go get yourself a drink of water" then it is to stop whatever you're doing and construct a sippy cup.

Make sure that plastic cups are safely within kids' reach. Also show them how to operate the sink so that they can get themselves water either from the tap or from a filtered water tap. Teach them to put the cup by the sink when they're done.

5. Children three-years-old throw out their trash in the house or car.

Juice boxes, candy wrappers, tissues, apple sauce or pudding cups, apple cores, and banana peels are a few examples of what kids can throw out themselves. Explain that when finished these items go in the trash. Give them what they need to succeed by making sure the trash receptacles in your home and car are accessible and easy to use. The "no one leaves the car empty-handed" rule applies here. Teach your kids to gather and throw out their trash before they leave the vehicle. See more time saving car tips in Chapter Six "Quick and Easy Family Travel"

6. Children three-years-old wash and dry their hands.

This is something kids do before every meal and after using the bathroom; therefore, teaching them how to do it on their own saves parents lots of time. Make sure the faucet they use is easy to turn on and off, and a towel is within reach. Also, don't forget to put a footstool in the bathroom, so they can reach the sink.

> *Placing a liquid soap dispenser at each sink makes hand washing easier for kids.*

7. Children three-years-old prepare a simple snack for themselves like an apple or banana.

"Mommy, I'm hungry!" I hear this from my kids four or five times a day. If kids know how to fix a simple snack for themselves, then they will when you permit. Keep nonperishable fruit such as apples or bananas on your kitchen table. Show your kids how to peel a banana and wash an apple. Make sure they have access to a footstool, so they can reach a sink. My kids wash their apples at the same tap they use to brush their teeth and wash their hands. If you prefer, pre-wash the apples before you set them out but remember—the point is to make less work for you by making your kids more self-reliant. My three- and five-year-olds wash their own apples.

8. Children three-years or older use the TV remote control to turn the TV on/off and tune in favorite channels.

Wouldn't it be great if your kids could tune in their favorite channels while you're feeding baby or taking a nap? Show them how.

9. Children four-years-old put dirty dishes by the sink.

10. Children two-and-a-half-years old play in a single room and clean up their toys.

When I was seven months pregnant, I couldn't see well below

me. I tripped over some toys on the dining room floor and broke my toe.

Toy clutter throughout the home not only makes it difficult to get from here to there; it's dangerous. Tripping, falling, and stepping on toys causes injury. Even more so after baby arrives because being tired and walking holding baby makes it hard to see what's beneath you. Moreover, with toys scattered about the home, it's more difficult to cleanup like vacuuming, dusting, and putting away laundry.

> *The best way to prevent toy clutter is to contain toys to a single room of the home.*

The best way to prevent toy clutter is to contain all toys to a single room of the home. If no one room is large enough, then each child's room can be used with toys restricted to those rooms only. Store toys within the room you designate, and show your kids where to put them away. If you use toy boxes, bins, basket, a closet, or shelves, then they should be within the room where the toys are played.

In our home, the designated toy room is the living room. Toys are stored in plastic bins and the floor of a living room coat closet for larger toys. There are no toys in the kids' bedrooms, only bookcases with books to read. Reading, quiet contemplation, and "time out" are done in their rooms; playtime is either in the backyard or living room. If they take a toy to another room of the house, they are reminded that they need to play with it in the living room. When the living room gets messy with toys, I simply tell my kids to clean it up. They know where everything goes.

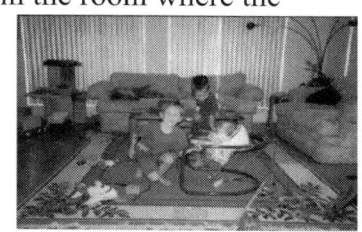

Toy play stays in living room.

Explain to your kids which room is for play and that toys are not to be removed. Tell them why, for example, toy clutter is dangerous and makes cleaning difficult. I've found that kids are more cooperative if they understand why they should or should not do something.

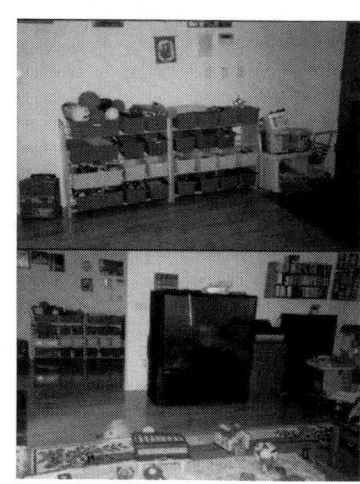

Toy bins by living room.

Eiche surprised me recently when we were at his friend's house. There were toys scattered about the hallway, on the stairs, and in the dining area, with the highest concentration of toys in the living room and kids' rooms. Eiche and his friend started to climb the stairs when his friend stepped on a toy and began crying. Eiche comforted him saying, "That's why you have to pick up your toys, because you can get hurt." My son follows our family's toy rules because he understands the reasons why we have toy rules.

> *Kids are much more cooperative if they understand the reasons why they should or shouldn't do something.*

Chapter Four

REDUCE TIME SPENT ON BILLS AND APPOINTMENTS

1. Hang a wall calendar for appointments, loan/bill due dates, parties, and vacations.

2. Memorize your and your spouse's social security numbers.

3. Synchronize bill due dates.

4. Pay bills automatically.

5. Pay bills online that cannot be paid automatically.

6. Manage your bank account via phone and laptop

7. Buy a set of assorted greeting cards for occasions.

8. Select and order birth announcements now.

9. Buy "thank you" cards, formal and informal.

10. Use a bank with drive-thru teller or ATM.

11. Direct deposit paychecks.

12. Use a post office with drive-thru.

13. Order postage stamps and return address labels online.

Everyone wants to spend as little time as possible paying bills, filling out forms, corresponding, or going to appointments. Once baby arrives, however, your time will be limited making these tasks more painful. Organization is key to efficiently and effectively managing these obligations. Reviewing bills, calling or emailing creditors, appointments, check writing, loan applications, filling out forms, filing statements and receipts typically take more than 15 minutes of uninterrupted concentration. That means it's a chore best done with baby asleep. Since baby sleep time is parent free time, these tasks cut into the little free time new parents have. You owe your creditors money not your time. Showing you ways to keep as much of your time yours by not giving it to creditors, appointments, forms, filing and correspondence is the focus of this chapter.

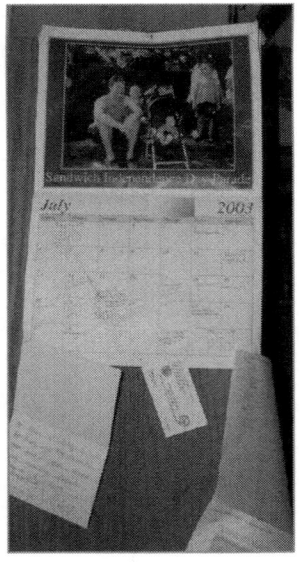

Party invitation, appointment card, and school field trip directions stapled to the bottom.

1. Hang a wall calendar for appointments, loan/bill due dates, parties, and vacations.

This is an easy way to get a grip on all your important dates. When you make an appointment, mark it on a calendar along with the phone number and address; that way if you have to cancel or call for directions, you're not running around looking for the phone number five minutes before you're supposed to be there. If you make an appointment when you're out of the house, write it down on a business card or take a photo of the business card with your phone. Once home, mark it on the calendar. If you need the business card for directions or instructions, staple it to the bottom of that month's calendar page. Do the same for all invitations requiring RSVP or have directions or instructions. When the day of the engagement arrives, simply tear the business card or invitation from the bottom of the calendar, follow the instructions or take it with you.

Be sure to mark any hefty or unusual bill due dates on your

calendar to avoid penalties and interest. I calendar the last possible day to pay my property taxes because I want to avoid the steep 10% penalty. I also calendar all credit card bills whose due dates are not synchronized with my other bills. Don't forget to mark any obligation that would prevent you from scheduling an appointment for a given day, such as vacations, grocery delivery, and so on.

One big benefit to using a wall calendar is that it provides a permanent record of what you did, with whom, and when. At the end of the year, store it with other old calendars. In later months or years, if you need to look up when you did something or with whom, just pull out your old calendars to look it up. Super handy. Has saved my bacon a number of times.

> *If you have trouble remembering relatives' birth dates and anniversaries, consider ordering a calendar with those dates preprinted.*

2. Memorize you and your spouse's social security numbers.

This information is easily memorized and frequently needed to prove identity, for medical care, insurance, bills, day care providers, loans, and so forth. Not knowing both numbers wastes time by looking for social security cards, repeatedly asking your spouse for their number, having to call someone back with the number, or when filling out forms.

> *Once you've memorized social security numbers, prevent identity theft by not carrying your social security card with you.*

3. Synchronize bill due dates.

Bill paying is time-consuming and unpleasant, so the less you have to do it the better. Most monthly bills are due around the first of the month. If you have bills that are due at other times, call vendors and request that due dates be changed to the first of the month. This way payment deadlines are easier to remember, and more bills can be paid together at one time—saving time and avoiding late fees and interest charges. If a vendor can't change a monthly due date, then request automatic pay (see items 5 and 6) or calendar the date so it's not missed.

Most creditors and banks allow you to set up automatic payment of your bills free of charge.

4. Pay bills automatically.

Set up online autopay for your bills. Then your only responsibility each month will be to review your statements for inaccuracies. Most creditors give you the opportunity to negotiate any charges with which you don't agree before automatic payment is made.

5. Pay bills online that cannot be paid automatically.

Some creditors offer online payment instead of autopay where you sign in and pay your bill each month, but the sorting, stuffing, addressing, and stamping of traditional paper bills are avoided.

TIP: Be cautious entering financial information online. Make sure your browser and the vendor's website are secure.

6. Manage your bank account via phone and laptop.

Access your bank account online, so you can review it for balance and check clearing information. You can transfer money between internal and external accounts. You can fill out loan applications online, or if you have a loan, then you can transfer payments to it.

Set up automatic monthly payment with your bank of any loans you have there.

7. Buy a set of assorted greeting cards.

Buy a set of assorted greeting cards for birthdays, holidays, baby showers, get well, and so on.

8. Select and order birth announcements before baby arrives.

Create online birth announcements to go paperless with free email delivery. Google for vendors. Or if you prefer paper announcements, vendors will let you select and order ahead even though you don't know details like gender or date of birth. Once you place your order, they'll send you envelopes to address now. When baby arrives, simply phone missing information into the vendor, and they will process the rest of your order. Once you receive the announcements, all you'll have to do is stuff envelopes and mail. For an added fee, some vendors will do the entire process of addressing, stuffing, and mailing.

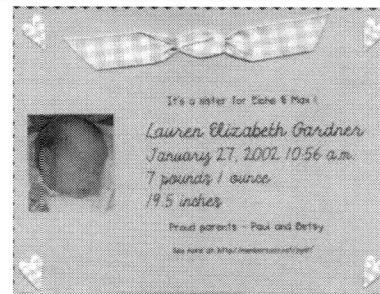

Make baby's picture part of announcement, so you won't need to add a separate photo.

10. Buy "thank you" cards, formal and informal.

Baby gifts come with babies. Be prepared to send appropriate "thank you" cards.

11. Use a bank with a drive-up teller or ATM.

If your bank does not offer drive-up service then consider switching to one that does. Getting children in and out of a vehicle is a time-consuming hassle that should be avoided as much as possible. To that end, drive-up banking is a terrific time saver. For more, see Chapter Six "Quick and Easy Family Travel."

12. Arrange direct deposit of paychecks.

Taking advantage of direct deposit, if offered by your employer, will save you trips to the bank.

TIP: Consider purchasing a computer address label program so you can print address labels for announcements, invitations, or holiday cards.

13. Use a post office with drive-thru.

Call your local U.S. post offices and see if any have a drive-thru window. If so, ask its hours and what postal business can be conducted. A post office near my home installed a drive-thru within the last two years and it has been a real life-saver in terms of managing my time. I can mail small packages, weigh envelopes to determine postage, buy stamps, and so forth without leaving my vehicle.

14. Order postage stamps and return address labels via the Web.

The U.S. Postal Service offers a number of items for sale through its website including stamps; visit https://www.usps.com for more information. Return address labels are useful not only for addressing envelopes but also for any situation in which your address is needed including filling in forms. Search the web for vendors.

Chapter Five

KEEP CAR TRIPS TO A MINIMUM

1. Order groceries online.

2. Order clothes, gifts, and more online.

3. Do as much banking and bill paying online as possible.

Time to grocery shop with the kids. Okay load backpack, diaper bag, juice, wipes, snacks, toys into the car. Next, put on shoes and jackets, negotiate car seats, dole out juice, snacks, and toys. Once there, renegotiate the car seats, make sure shoes and jackets are still on, unload infant car seat carrier, and have everyone hold hands crossing the parking lot.

Finally, time to shop. Hmm, what kind of bread do you need? But wait! The kids are running around the aisles. Baby is crying and needs soothing. Okay, you get your kids under control, hold the baby, and reconsider your choices. But wait! One kid wants coupons from the coupon machine in the aisle and another wants a cereal with a toy surprise. Hold it! Remember you turned your back? Are all your kids still with you? Okay yes, 1, 2, 3 they're all here. Now what were you thinking about? Oh yeah, what kind of bread to buy. But wait! Now your son needs to go to the bathroom. Can he hold it? No, he insists he can't. Locate the bathroom. Leave your cart outside and bring all the kids with you inside. Now your daughter says she has to go too. Help the two kids go to the bathroom while holding baby. Everyone wash hands and dry too. Okay, back to the cart.

Done shopping at last and time to check out. Uh oh, there's a candy display in the checkout lane. You quickly scan the other lanes. Yes, they all have them. The kids are begging for candy. The line is long and the cashier is slow. Why do you always pick the slowest line? The baby is crying again. The items are scanned, and you insert your debit card. But wait! You were busy talking to the cashier. Are all your kids still with you? One is missing! Okay, it's okay; there she is over by the toy vending machine next to the automatic doors. Better keep an eye on her to make sure she doesn't wander out.

Time to go home. Everyone hold hands in the parking lot. Load the infant car seat into the car. Get the other kids into their car seats. Load up the groceries. Drive home. Renegotiate the car seats yet again. Herd everyone into the house. Tend to baby. Unload and put away the groceries. Whew! Don't you wish there was an easier, safer, and less stressful way to grocery shop? There is.

1. Order groceries online.

When I suggest Internet grocery delivery to busy parents, their five main concerns are: (1) *quality*, the freshness of meat and produce; (2) *cost*, the price of delivery; (3) *security*, the safety of their bank information; (4) *ease of website ordering*, the website be easy to use; and (5) *availability*, delivery services their area. Let's address these concerns.

Quality. When I began investigating grocery delivery, I was skeptical. Would the food be fresh? Would it be the quality I'd select myself? Could I still buy all my favorite foods? I discovered that freshness and selection varied by delivery services. I selected a service a few months before my second son was born which had high quality food and almost every item I wanted. It's much easier to grocery shop once every few months for those one or two items that are missing than to shop each week for everything we need.

> *If you only have two days off a week to spend with your family, then grocery shopping on one of those days costs the family most dearly in family time.*

Cost. Some people don't like paying for grocery delivery because they don't like paying for something that they can do themselves for "free." What they fail to consider, however, is that conventional grocery shopping is not free. As I briefly illustrated at the beginning of this chapter, there's the value of your time and sanity. It's particularly valuable in families where both parents work outside the home. If you only have two days off a week to spend with your family, then grocery shopping on one of those days costs the family most dearly in family time. Additionally, if you're traveling to the grocery store more than once a week for forgotten items, then it's costing you even greater time and aggravation.

If you still think grocery delivery is too expensive, consider this: a meal at a fast-food restaurant for a family of four (or two large pizzas) is about $20, more than the standard $10 grocery delivery fee (some grocery delivery fees are even lower, $5 to $9). If you eat out with your family one less time a month, you've paid for the cost of grocery delivery, and if you have your groceries delivered, you're much less likely to forget something making it less likely that you'll need to take the family out to eat. Why are you less likely to forget something? Because with grocery delivery, you order from your home without the distraction of kids in a store, and you can look in your kitchen when ordering to see what you need.

> *Online shopping is safer for your kids because there's no chance of losing them in a store or a stranger luring them away.*

Security. Some people think ordering over the Web is unsafe. They worry that their credit card or other personal information will fall into the wrong hands. This is an understandable concern that can be addressed by prudent shopping. Be as cautious on the internet as you would in a regular store. Buy from reputable grocery chains and delivery services. Such establishments have secure websites.

By focusing on money alone, parents often forget about the safety of their most important asset—their children. Let's put security in perspective. Undeniably, Web shopping is safer for kids because there's no chance of losing them in a store, or a stranger luring them away.

> *If your browser does not show a "lock" graphic, do not enter your financial information.*

Ease of online ordering. Websites are designed to make grocery shopping easy and familiar with pictures of products and a shopping cart. If you shop with a grocery list, simply take it to your computer instead of a store. If you don't use a list, then simply take yourself to your computer rather than a store. I once suggested online grocery shopping to a tired and busy mom who told me she hadn't tried it because she "can't plan meals ahead." I asked her if she took a grocery list with her shopping. "Always," she responded. "Isn't it easier to take your grocery list to your computer than to a grocery store?" I asked.

Searching online for items is easier than searching for them at a supermarket because of keyword searching. Simply type in what you're looking for, e.g., "banana," hit return and all types available are displayed within seconds. No more dragging your kids up and down aisles to find something.

Additionally, what you bought in the past is available as a list to order from every time you shop. This makes preparing your favorite meals quick and easy because once ingredients are purchased, they remain on your online grocery list for future selection. Just choose an item once for your grocery cart without searching for it ever again.

Availability. Most areas are serviced by a grocery delivery company. Some areas are serviced by more than one. Search the Web or call your local grocery stores to find out who offers this service. The following is a list of things to consider when selecting a service for grocery delivery.

> *Searching on grocery websites is even easier the second time you shop because purchased items stay on your online list for future orders.*

(1) The delivery schedule, how soon after the order is placed can they deliver? Do they have convenient delivery times?
(2) Delivery cost?
(3) Can you change your order before delivery? This is important because it's easy to forget items even when you order from home. Most delivery services allow you to add or subtract from your order up until the driver has left.
(4) Is the website easy to use? How difficult is it to navigate to the items you want to buy? How easy and secure is it to pay online?
(5) Do they offer a wide variety of foods as well as toiletries, over the counter medicines, baby care items?
(6) Are meat and produce fresh?
(7) Is the service good? Did they deliver on time? Was the delivery person professional? Did you get everything you ordered? If there were brand or item substitutions, were they acceptable.
(8) Do they offer good customer service? Is there a phone number or email if you're not happy? How long does it take them to respond? Did they readily credit your account or did you have to argue for credit?
(9) Do they accept coupons?

One of the newest options for grocery delivery is crowdsource picking and delivering. Crowdsource is a service model started by taxi-like services Uber and Lyft. Grocery delivery companies like Instacart (and its competitors) use the internet to vet and register a large group of people to shop and deliver groceries. You can pay per delivery (about $10), or you can purchase a yearly membership (about $99). Delivery is free with membership as long as you purchase a minimum of $25 worth of groceries (easy to do these days with things being so expensive). There's a default tip of 5%, but you don't have to tip anything, or you can tip more. There are a lot of advantages to Instacart. First, they don't run out of delivery times due to the large pool of people available to shop and deliver. Second, your grocery shopper is careful about what they select because they want a good tip. Third, your shopper communicates with you via text while they select your items making it easy for you to change or add to your order as they shop. Fourth, your shopper lets you know via text when they finish shopping, so you know when they are on the way to your door.

There are many things I enjoy about online groceries, for instance, no traveling, hauling grocery bags, arguing with the kids. If I'm interrupted, I can return to finish entering my order later. I find items quickly without dragging kids up and down grocery aisles. No more waiting in long checkout lines with kids drooling over candy displays. I can order late at night, early in the morning, in my pajamas, or anytime. There's one advantage to it, however, which I cannot get over—ordering from my kitchen. When I can't remember if I have enough flour or milk or juice or whatever, all I have to do is take literally six steps to the pantry or refrigerator and look. How cool is that?

2. Order clothes, gifts and more online.

Going clothes shopping with kids in tow is as time-consuming and aggravating as grocery shopping. More, if you try clothes on. Kids running around the changing room and peeking into stalls as you race to undress, dress, undress, and dress. Do you want to spend your time doing this? I simply cannot. I cannot try clothes on with two kids and a baby. I've tried. It's just not possible to watch over them and undress, dress, consider my options, make a purchasing decision, then undress and dress again What's a busy parent to do? Voila, online shopping! No more hauling the kids to the store. No more embarrassing peep show incidents in the changing rooms. No more playing hide and seek in the display racks. No more looking for discreet places to change and feed baby. No more shopping in terror of hearing, "Mommy, I have to go to the bathroom!" And, don't forget the most important advantage of all—safety—no chance of losing your child in the store.

Choices for online shopping include Amazon, Walmart, JCPenney, Macy's, Nordstrom, Walmart, Target, Old Navy, Gap, Lowes, Home Depot, and more. Check with local retailers or google for availability. In addition to offering a secure site for payment, retailers offer fair return policies. Amazon makes it super easy to return things. Login and click "return" and Amazon emails you a QR code. Bring your return to any UPS Store. They scan the QR code from your phone, and pack and ship your item for free. Experiment with online ordering and returns before baby arrives.

QR Code

When I suggest online clothes shopping to busy parents, their biggest concerns are buying clothes that don't fit and the cost of delivery. However, I've found it easier to buy the right clothing size when you shop online because the size charts are more detailed than a clothing tag and pop up with a click of your mouse.

If you limit clothes and other shopping to secure online sites run by reputable chains, then the only other concern is cost. What are your time and energy worth? Is it worth the cost of delivery? Whether or not the amount is reasonable will vary from person to person, but consider these examples. I purchased nine shirts for myself from JCPenney online. The entire transaction including selection and purchase took 20 minutes. The cost of delivery was free because the store had an anniversary sale that included free shipping. If I had gone to the store, travel time would've been 30 minutes and shopping time 1 hour at my local JCPenney with two kids and a baby which totals 1.5 hours, maybe more if one of my kids has to use the bathroom, or I have to stop to feed or change the baby. By shopping online, I bought myself an hour and ten

> *It's easier to buy the right clothing size on the Internet because the size charts are more detailed than a clothing tag and "pop up" with the click of a mouse.*

minutes with no aggravation, no exhaustion, and no additional cost. Worth it?

Let's take another example. I purchased 13 baby clothing items, for example, tops, body suits, leggings, shorts, and five pairs of shorts for my two older kids. The entire purchase took about 30 minutes; longer than the Penney's purchase because I had to consult online size charts and order for three different kids. The shipping cost was $11.95. My local Old Navy is 40 minutes total travel time. The time to shop for three kids with them along would be about 1.5 hours because I cannot take shopping with them any longer than that. Total time would be at least 2 hours and 10 minutes, so for $11.95, I bought myself at least an hour and 40 minutes. Worth it?

Let's consider one more example. I bought puzzles for my kids from Walmart. My kids love puzzles. The purchase took 15 minutes. The shipping cost was $7.83. My local Walmart is a 30-minute drive. As any parent knows, and others of you will soon discover, shopping for toys is an especially stressful and time-consuming outing. Excited kids run around demanding toys and throwing temper tantrums. Total time would therefore be 1 hour and 30 minutes—longer if I had to take kids to the bathroom or change and feed baby, so for $7.83, I bought myself 1 hour and 30 minutes. Worth it?

Other time-saving advantages to shopping online: keyword search for an item is easier than running up and down store aisles, review your account to track packages, your purchase history is kept at most sites for at least two months and at others for years to review whenever you wish, and register your credit card information for quick checkout.

How about shopping for a baby shower gift? Anniversary gift? Birthday gift? Housewarming gift? Holiday gift? Okay, prepare the diaper bag, load the stroller, put jackets on the kids, herd them into the car, secure them in their car seats, dole out the juice and snacks, and drive...*stop!* Buying gifts online is easier for you and safer for your kids. Also, for a small fee most sites will gift wrap for you and ship direct. That's a real time saver! Evaluate shipping, wrapping, and return charges versus time saved and decide for yourself whether it's a worthy purchase.

3. Do as much banking and bill paying online as possible.

There's one important time savings relevant here; namely, that you travel to the bank or post office as little as possible. Set up automatic bill payment with your creditors, set up paycheck direct deposit, and so forth. See Chapter Four "Reduce Time Spent On Bills and Appointments" for a complete discussion of how this saves time.

Chapter Six

QUICK AND EASY FAMILY TRAVEL

1. Buy a car seat for your infant or toddler that's easy to use.

2. Purchase seats for older children that they can secure themselves.

3. Use a backpack diaper bag.

4. Use a drive-thru pharmacy.

5. Use a drive-thru bank teller or ATM.

6. Use a post office with a drive-thru window.

7. Everyone in the car is responsible for their own trash.

8. Teach kids "The Empty-Hand Rule": No one gets in or out of the car empty handed.

To save time and energy, you've done everything possible to avoid using your vehicle. See Chapter Five "Keep Car Trips to a Minimum"; nevertheless, there are times when you must go out. With kids, getting in and out of a car is a real chore. If you're awaiting the arrival of your first child then you may be thinking, "How hard can it be?" Consider the car seat, stroller, backpack, diaper bag, and other baby gear you've been buying. That's a lot of gear for a lot of work! Fortunately, there are ways to make it easier to get in and out of your vehicle, as well as reduce the number of times you need to. Here's how.

1. Buy a car seat for your infant or toddler that's easy to use.

Car seats are lifesaving devices that safeguard our precious children. We use them because we love and want to protect them. But let's be honest, using car seats is an ordeal especially if you have two or more kids in them at once.

Consider how much you're repeatedly doing with car seats: lifting and carrying infant seats, lifting of toddlers into and out of, reminding older kids to climb into their seat, buckling and unbuckling a four-point restraint or booster seatbelt, aligning or adjusting a seatbelt guide clip, etc. Regardless of how your car seat functions, you're performing these tasks each time you get in and out of your car. The hoisting of kids including car seat fastening and unfastening takes a toll on parents physically. If your vehicle is a car, then you're stooping over to lift into, fasten, unfasten, and lift out. If your vehicle is a van, SUV, or truck, then you're lifting up to, fasten, unfasten, and lift out. Moreover, with a van or SUV, you're climbing into the back to secure kids. No wonder parents are tired!

> *A well-designed car seat should be easy to use.*

A car seat can be a daily source of anger, frustration, and anxiety. Spend time now purchasing one that's easy to use, and you'll reap daily dividends in time and energy. If you're shopping for an infant or toddler seat, try it out in the store. Is it easy to get baby or toddler in and out? Is it easy for you to fasten and unfasten? When you purchase a seat, hold on to the receipt for 30 days. Follow the manufacturer's installation and use instructions and put the car seat on trial. A well-designed seat should be easy to use. If after thirty days you're not happy with its ease of use, then return it and put a different one on thirty-day trial.

2. Purchase seats for older children that they can secure themselves.

Consult your state's laws for requirements regarding car seats for kids. Most children don't fit properly in seatbelts until at least age eight, so the bottom line is that you'll be tending to kids in car seats for *years,* and the older your kids get while using car seats, the more likely it is that they'll become smart enough and physically capable enough to release themselves from their restraint either fully or partially.

It's a lot easier for older children (four years or more) to release themselves from a car seat then it is for them to secure themselves. Why? Because often, releasing is as easy as pressing a button on a buckle. If it's a seatbelt run through a car seat's guide clip, then the belt is under tension and simply releases and retracts once the car's seatbelt release button is pressed. If it's a four-point restraint seat, once pressed, the release button releases the bottom two points of the four-point restraint harness—the other two points are held by a guide clip that children have difficulty unfastening, so releasing all or part of the restraint is fairly easy for kids once they reach the right stage of intelligence and dexterity.

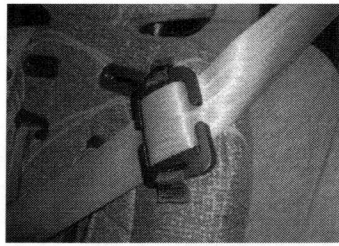

Most kids cannot get the seatbelt through the guide clip themselves, and in those seats in which the seat belt remains in the clip at all times, pulling the seatbelt to create enough slack to run it across their body is difficult.

Although unfastening their car seat is easy for older children, securing themselves is not because of car seat guide clips. In most car seats for kids over 40 pounds, the seatbelt must be run through a guide clip that positions the seatbelt properly over the child's shoulder. Most kids cannot get the seatbelt through the guide themselves, and in those seats in which the seatbelt remains in the clip at all times, pulling the seatbelt to create enough slack to run it across their body is difficult. The clip tends to hold the belt tight, and most children simply cannot stretch the belt long enough to buckle it, and in the four-point restraint car seat, the top two points of restraint are a guide clip. The only way for a child to get into the restraint is to put their arms under the restraint belts, and then clip them with the guide clip. This is simply too difficult for most children.

Consider this: if your child already knows how to release their car seat, then doesn't it make sense to buy them a seat in which they can also *secure* themselves? When I was expecting my third child, I faced a dilemma: my five-year-old would have to move to the back seat of the van to make room for the baby, but I didn't want to go back there with him! He had the ability to unbuckle his car seat himself, but due to a guide clip in the shoulder area he was unable to buckle it. Even though he was able to release himself from his car seat, he knew it was important that he remain secured while driving, and he did.

Since I felt he was ready, I bought him a high back booster seat that I thought he'd be able to get in and out of himself. Even though the birth of the baby was three months away, we moved my son to the back seat and installed the booster. After thirty days, we found that he still could not manage the seat because the seatbelt kept slipping out of its guide clip. He

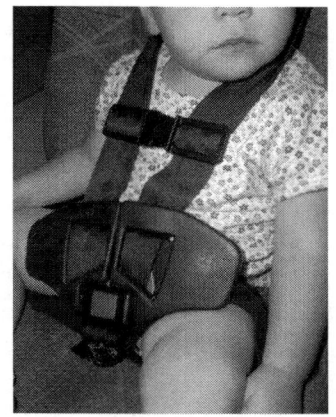

Four-point restraint has a guide clip as the upper two points and a buckle as the lower two points. Most kids age four and over can release the bottom two points by simply pressing the release button. Most cannot fasten or release the guide clip upper two points.

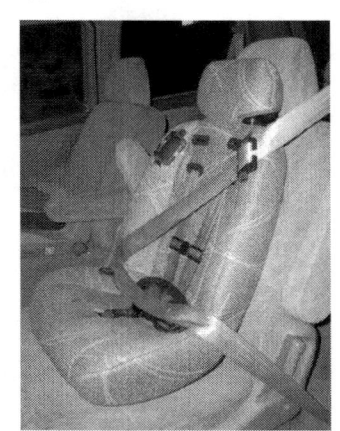

When the child reaches the height and weight indicated by the car seat manufacturer, they can use the car seat with a shoulder "guide clip." The child is secured by the car's seatbelt run through the guide clip.

simply could not put the belt back through himself, so I returned it. I bought another booster, this time backless. It went on thirty-day trial and passed. My son was able to buckle and unbuckle the seatbelt properly. When the baby came, I didn't have to worry about getting him in and out of the van because he could do it himself.

At this time, I also had a three-and-a-half-year-old son who weighed 40 pounds. He sat in a car seat behind me and next to where the baby would soon sit. He had a four-point restraint car seat and could release the buckle or bottom two-point restraint (but not the top two-point guide clip). When he saw his older brother move to the back seat and learn to buckle and unbuckle his own booster, then he wanted to do it too. He wanted to be a "big boy." I double checked the manufacturer's instructions, verified my son's weight and height, and discovered that he could use the same booster, so I bought another and installed it. My three-and-a-half-year-old had more difficulty than my older son at first, but after thirty days we found that he could also buckle and unbuckle the seat. He too remained secure while driving and did not unbuckle the car seat when the car was in motion, so we told him he could continue using the new booster seat. When the baby came, the only child I had to fasten in and out of a car seat was the baby.

If you have a child between the ages of three and four, you've probably had to remind them to keep their car seat fastened while driving. If you find that

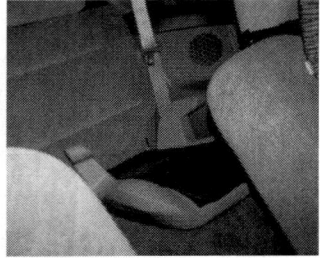

Booster seat for my five-year-old son. According to the manufacturer, backless boosters such as these are only to be used in vehicles with high back seats. This booster is for children who are 40 to 80 pounds and whose seated height places the midpoint of the head below the top of the car seat's backrest or whose standing height is 60 inches (152 cm) or less. If the seatbelt does not lie correctly across the shoulder, then a shoulder belt clip, provided by the manufacturer with the car seat, must be used.

> *You'll be tending to kids in car seats for years. If your child is old enough to fully or partially release themselves from their car seat, doesn't it make sense to buy them one in which they can also secure themself?*

they do in fact stay buckled up even though they may be able to partially or fully unbuckle themselves, then they may be ready for a car seat that they can both get into and out of by themselves. When purchasing such a car seat, keep the receipt, follow the manufacturer's installation and use instructions, and put the seat on thirty-day trial. If by the end of that time your child cannot get into the seat, fasten and unfasten it properly without help, then return it.

> *Keep an extra booster or car seat in the trunk for play dates. This way when friends want to come over after school, you can drive them safely and legally.*

Let me be clear here. I care about the safety of you and your kids. If your child will not remain secured in their car seat when riding in the car then buy him or her a seat that he or she cannot get out of. It's your responsibility as their parent to make certain that your child stays properly secured in their car seat while the car is in motion. Remember also, **if your kids are securing themselves into car seats, it's your responsibility to check and make sure they are properly securing themselves every single time they use them.** Before starting my car, I ask if everyone is buckled up and I turn around to look at my kids and *see* that they are properly secured in their car seats.

3. Use a backpack diaper bag.

A backpack diaper bag saves time because it leaves your hands free. With hands free, you can hold baby, hold your kids' hands in parking lots, talk on your cell phone while carrying baby, carry things back and forth to your car, etc. Shoulder diaper bags, on the other hand, slip off and causes neck and shoulder pain. Look for a backpack diaper bag that has a built-in changing pad that folds out from the side—super convenient, no more searching the bag for the changing pad.

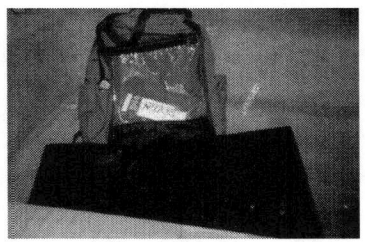

Backpack diaper bag features a built-in changing pad that unfolds from the side.

Another great feature of a backpack diaper bag is that it's more masculine and so more acceptable to Dad. Since Dad will be doing half the diaper changes or more, it's a good idea to buy a diaper bag he's comfortable with.

4. Use a drive-thru pharmacy.

Kids get sick a lot. They bring colds home with them from playdates, preschool, elementary school, and after-school activities. It's also common for baby, mom or both to need prescriptions filled after birth. Large pharmacies have drive-thru windows. Call pharmacies in your area to find one. Switch your prescriptions over to that pharmacy now before baby arrives. Beyond saving time, it's a relief not dragging sick kids out of the car. Also, if you ask nicely, a pharmacy drive-thru will also sell nonprescription children's medicine such as infant or children's flu formula, cough suppressant, and so on.

> *Carry your pharmacy phone number with you. When you need a prescription filled, give it to your pediatrician to phone in. Then all you have to do is pick it up.*

5. Use a drive-thru bank teller or ATM.

The less you have to get your kids out of the car the better. Although a lot of banking can be done online, some transactions like making deposits or getting cash cannot. If your bank doesn't offer drive-thru service, then consider switching to one that does.

6. Use a post office with a drive-thru window.

Using a postal drive-up window also expedites bill paying. For more, see Chapter Four "Minimize Time Spent on Bill Payment and Appointments."

7. Everyone in the car is responsible for their own trash.

It's easier to get in and out of an uncluttered vehicle. Keep a supply of plastic grocery bags in your car for use as trash bags. Whenever a member of the family has trash in the car, like an empty juice box or food wrapper, they know it's their responsibility to throw it out.

8. Teach kids "The Empty-Hand Rule": No one gets in or out of the car empty handed.

Teach your kids that no one gets in or out of the car without something. If kids have coats, jackets, shoes, backpacks, cell phone or whatever, it is their responsibility to take it in and out of the car. See more in Chapter Three "Siblings Are Self-Reliant." If they have nothing to bring in or take out of the car, then they can help dad and mom carry bags, baby toys, and so on. With praise, even kids as young as two years are eager and proud to help mom and dad.

Chapter Seven

FAST AND FRUSTRATION FREE COOKING WITH BABY

1. Make your brood the same food.

2. Limit breakfast and lunch choices and rotate.

3. Think about what to make for dinner once a week.

4. Keep dinner preparation 15 minutes or less with time-saving ingredients

5. Make more dinner than needed without adding preparation time.

6. Save leftovers.

7. No special orders ever.

8. Buy help yourself snacks.

The 15-minute baby contentment window after feeding and diaper change doesn't leave parents much time to prepare breakfast, lunch, or dinner; however, if you shop and cook with that time limit in mind, it's enough. The secret is to make meals that require either a total preparation time of 15 minutes, or 15 minutes of preparation to set it baking, grilling, microwaving, simmering, or boiling. This chapter shows you how.

> *If you don't have enough of the same thing for everyone, then don't make it. This prevents arguments and tantrums. Making the brood the same food saves cleanup and preparation time.*

1. Make your brood the same food.

To save time, make your kids the same thing. That way, for example, you only have to get out the bologna rather than the bologna, ham, and peanut butter and jelly. Remember too, everything you take out has to be put back, so making the brood the same food saves cleanup time too. It also prevents arguments, changed minds, jealousy, temper tantrums, and fights. If one child has bologna and the other ham, inevitably one will want what the other has, and to further avoid meltdowns, if you don't have enough of the same thing for everyone, then don't make it.

> *For sandwiches, store an extra loaf of bread in your freezer, so you don't run out. A few seconds in the microwave quickly thaws slices.*

2. Limit breakfast, lunch choices and rotate.

Traditionally, breakfast and lunch are individual meals made separately like cereal, bagel or sandwich. Dinner, on the other hand, is prepared as a large offering for family to share when they come together at the end of the day.

    I developed a system that turns the individual meal which is the basis of breakfast and lunch to your advantage. How? By limiting what to make for breakfast and lunch and putting those selections on rotation. To be clear, this is not a menu of options from which kids choose. If I opened the choice up to the kids, there'd be arguing. These are options for me to make, and I decide; for example, I limit the possibilities for lunch to three or four. The lunch choices take no more than 15 minutes to prepare which is within the baby contentment window. In my home right now, the lunch choices are ham sandwich, bologna sandwich, and peanut butter and jelly. I rotate these three selections throughout the week. One day it's ham, the next it's P.B. & J., the next it's bologna, and so forth. This way I don't waste time wondering what to make, and the ingredients are easily remembered when creating a grocery list. I add tasty, nutritious side dishes to lunch if they're no more effort than opening a package and placing on a plate, for instance, cheese sticks, pickles, apple sauce cups, or yogurt. Serve with milk or juice. There are plenty of prepackaged lunch items that parents can consider for rotation too such as frozen mini-pizzas, macaroni and cheese, and so on.

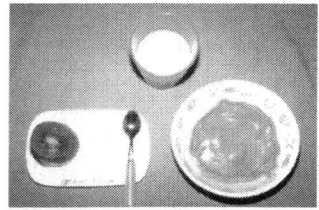

Microwave scrambled egg with cheese in a ceramic bowl is great by itself or in a breakfast sandwich. Also shown, easy kiwi. Sliced off end allows kids to eat it like a hardboiled egg. Provide a small spoon to scoop the meat out of the skin.

    Treat breakfast like lunch. Limit the choices to three or four and put them on rotation. Currently, the breakfast rotation in my home is frozen waffle, scrambled egg with a slice of cheese, and donut. Include a fruit side dish that's quick and easy, like a banana, strawberries, apple sauce cup, or kiwi. Today, for example, breakfast was microwave scrambled egg with cheese, kiwi, and milk. Cold cereal is also a quick and easy breakfast option, but if you're frustrated that

> *If you make lunches for school, then keep them on rotation too. For example, with one child in school and another at home, make the lunch for school and the one for home together. Store the home lunch in the refrigerator for lunchtime.*

your kids seem to like the sugary kind, then try offering it only if they finish the rest of their breakfast.

Put whatever meals you decide on breakfast and lunch rotation; just remember to select meals that are *quick and easy*, in other words, made within the 15-minute baby contentment window, and to serve everyone *the same thing*.

3. Think about what to make for dinner once a week.

When you wake, your first thoughts should be about the possibilities of the day—not the possibilities of your freezer. The solution? Think about what to make for dinner once a week on a night when you have a few minutes free. What I like to do is take a note pad and create a dinner menu and shopping list for the week or, as I call it a "dinner/shopping list."

Divide a sheet into left and right sides. On the left under "Menu," list the seven days of the week. Underneath each day write what you'll make for dinner. Then let your dinner menu on the left generate your shopping list on the right. If you don't have the ingredients, then write them down on the right side to know what to buy. Now when you wake up and go to the kitchen for coffee, all you'll have to do is look at the menu side of the list to see what's for dinner that night. If you don't feel like making or eating that particular meal, then simply switch it for another night's selection. If you need to take something out of the freezer to defrost, do it then. You won't worry about whether you have all the ingredients because you thought of them when you made the list, and you shopped from your list. If you decide that you want to go out for dinner that night, no problem; just shift the menu forward by a day and use it tomorrow. Because of this method, at my house we go out to dinner because we want to—not because we have to.

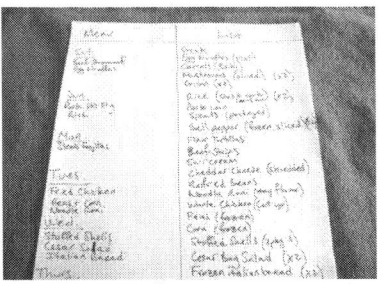

If you let your dinner menu generate your shopping list, you'll have the confidence to forget about dinner until it's time to make it.

Since there are only ten meals or so in my dinner repertoire, it takes me no more than 15 minutes to generate a weekly dinner/shopping list. If you let your dinner menu generate your shopping list and buy from your list, you'll have the confidence you need to forget about what to make for dinner. You only have to glance at the menu in the morning, take out something to defrost if necessary, and then forget about dinner until it's time to make it.

Once you've let your dinner menu generate a list, add items that you need for breakfast and lunch rotation as well as "help yourself" snacks. Don't forget to add general household maintenance products including cleaning supplies, toiletries, diapers, wipes, cosmetics, and so on. Save even more time and energy by taking your list to your computer and ordering online for delivery. See Chapter Five "Keep Car Trips to a Minimum" for more.

> *The secret to stress-free cooking with baby is to take advantage of the 15-minute baby contentment window. Make meals that require either a total preparation time of 15 min. or 15 min. of preparation to set cooking.*

These days, my first thoughts are about my new daughter's smile and when she'll awaken. I consider fun places to take my family. Simply put, my first thoughts are about the possibilities of the day not the possibilities of my freezer.

4. Keep dinner preparation 15 minutes or less with time-saving ingredients.

The secret to stress-free cooking with baby is to make dinner within the 15-minute baby contentment window. Unfortunately, however, a traditional sit-down, quality family dinner usually takes longer than 15 minutes to prepare. The solution? Select meals that require 15 minutes or less preparation time. If a recipe requires a total cooking time of 30 minutes, 45 minutes, 1 hour, or more, that's fine as long as it takes you no longer than 15 minutes to get the meal started and requires little or no attention while cooking. You want "set and forget" meals that you can quickly get started and forget about until they're done. If you change and feed baby just before starting to make dinner, then you

> *Preparing meals that take 15 minutes to start cooking does not require new recipes but does require making your current recipes with time-saving ingredients*

should have enough time to get it going. While it cooks, you can do other things like soothe baby, homework with your kids, or empty the dishwasher. And what if you find yourself with a baby that fusses seemingly nonstop and doesn't seem to have a contentment window? Well, doesn't that make it even more sensible to make meals as quickly as possible?

This does not require new recipes. It does require, however, that you prepare your current recipes with time-saving ingredients. Review your recipes to see if this will work. After reviewing my dinner recipes, I found that there were two that could not be changed so that they could be started within 15 minutes. I sped up the preparation of the remaining recipes by cooking with time-saving ingredients.

Time-saving ingredients are traditional dinner ingredients repackaged to save time. For instance, bell pepper is a common dinner ingredient used in fajitas, stir fry, and pasta dishes which is now available as bags of frozen pepper strips. These are bags of red, yellow, and green bell pepper pre-washed, seedless, and sliced into strips. Some varieties contain onion strips as well! Just open the bag and pour. Mushrooms used to be sold whole and unwashed; now they're available in boxes washed and sliced. Frozen chopped spinach is another real time saver. Cook it in the microwave and you can add it to stir fry, lasagna, and more. If you have recipes that need pressed or minced garlic, try using garlic salt or powder instead. Many dinner recipes require carrots. Did you know you can buy bags of baby carrots that are pre-skinned and washed? Moreover, baby carrots are small, eliminating the need to chop. Simply open the bag and pour them into the pot. Shredding cheese is a real time waster and mess creator. If a recipe requires shredded cheese, then buy it already shredded in a bag. Need chicken or beef stock for a recipe? Use a beef or chicken bouillon cube.

> *Chopping, slicing, washing, grating, straining, and pressing are the most time-consuming parts of making dinner. Shop with the goal of eliminating/reducing these actions, and you'll transform your favorite meals into "fast food."*

Here are some examples of dinners I made for my family before the baby came which I continue to make after because of time-saving ingredients. My point is to illustrate how you can make your favorite recipes more quickly and easily, **not to suggest new ones**. When you look at these examples, think about how these ingredients could be used in your own recipes to save time. On the left is the meal and on the right are the time-saving ingredients.

Four Pepper Pasta	1 bag frozen pepper strips, 1 box pre-washed and sliced mushrooms, garlic powder, dried minced onion.
Beef Stroganoff/Stew	1 box pre-washed and sliced mushrooms, 1 bag pre-washed baby carrots, garlic salt, dried minced onion, 1 pound package stew beef cubes.
Sizzling Steak Fajitas	1 bag frozen pepper strips, 1 can refried beans, 1 bag shredded cheddar cheese, 1 pound package beef strips.
Pot Roast	1 bag pre-washed baby carrots, dried minced onion.
Stir Fry	1 bag pre-washed baby carrots, 1 bag frozen pepper strips, 1 box pre-washed sprouts, 1 box pre-washed and sliced mushrooms, garlic powder.
Chef's Salad	1 bag pre-washed salad, 1 box pre-washed and sliced mushrooms, 1 box pre-washed sprouts, 1/8 bag pre-washed baby carrots, 1/4 bag

	shredded cheese.
Chicken Marsala	1 box pre-washed and sliced mushrooms, 1/2 bouillon cube, garlic powder.

These are meals that typically took thirty minutes or more to start, but by substituting time-saving ingredients I transformed them into fare that take 15 minutes or less to get cooking. Now I can walk away and do other things.

Evaluate your favorite home cooked dinners. Identify what part takes the longest to get them cooking. I've found that it's usually chopping, slicing, washing, grating, straining, or pressing. Shop with the goal of eliminating or reducing these actions during dinner preparation, and you'll find other ingredients that will transform your favorite meals into "fast food."

Of course, the ultimate time-saving ingredient is one that completely replaces dinner. Consider replacing dinners with packaged meals that are every bit as good as what you make. I'm serious. I consider myself a picky eater and will not eat anything that I can make better. When I began investigating replacement as a time-saving possibility, I wasn't hopeful. However, I've been pleasantly surprised by some of my discoveries. Take spaghetti sauce for example. There are lots of varieties; all of them are as good as homemade not some are. You'll save a ton of time but buying jar spaghetti sauce to use in spaghetti, lasagna, stuffed shells, and other Italian fare. Speaking of stuffed shells and lasagna, there are frozen food versions that are just excellent. I no longer make homemade stuffed shells and lasagna since what's available frozen is good. Even though they take thirty minutes or more to cook, all you have to do is pop in the oven and walk away.

> *Run hot water over frozen veggies in a strainer to thaw and reduce water prior to cooking.*

Fish is a meal that I thought I'd have to give up until baby was older because it's time-consuming to buy and prepare. I will only eat fresh fish which means either a trip to the market for fish to be cooked that day, or cooking fish that was delivered via online shopping on the day of delivery. Additionally, fish is difficult to prepare because it has to be deboned. Even though I'd never had frozen fish, I decided to give it a whirl. I sampled some packaged frozen fish filets and found a number of the breaded ones to be quite good. Since you can set them baking and forget until done, I added them to my dinner repertoire

> *It's handy to have a couple of pounds of ground beef in the freezer because it's so versatile. Use for hamburgers, sloppy joe, Hamburger Helper, pasta sauce.*

Side dishes can also be quick and easy. Packaged, pre-washed salad is an example. Pour it into a bowl and serve. Frozen Italian or garlic bread can be popped into the oven and ready in twenty minutes. Whether microwaved or cooked on a stove top, frozen corn, corn cobettes, peas, beans, or spinach require only pouring into a pot to cook. Canned vegetables are just as easily prepared. Frozen french fries are another great side dish that requires simply placing on a baking sheet to cook. Don't forget baked potato which you can easily microwave or bake. Rice is another good side that you can set cooking and forget until done. To save even more time, try some of the new five-minute rices in white, wild, and other varieties.

5. Make more dinner than needed without adding preparation time

Microwaving leftovers is a lot faster than cooking something new; therefore, if you can make more dinner than you need and still keep preparation time under 15 minutes, it will save you future time. Generate leftovers that you can use during the week as a quick lunch for yourself (unless you are on rotation with your kids) or to use again for dinner. When I prepare a large pot roast or baked chicken, I have plenty of main course leftovers; sometimes enough to eat for dinner a second time later in the week.

Leftovers repeatedly rescue me. I routinely make more than the family needs of corn, peas, beans, rice or whatever, so I have leftovers. Two or three nights later, I heat my leftover rice or corn or whatever and serve with the meal. It's easier and less costly than opening a new package. And, if a leftover side dish alone is not enough, I combine it with other leftovers to create a medley, for example, corn and peas, rice and corn, and so on.

> *If you have more than one child, consider purchasing a second microwave. With two you can cook dinner and heat a baby bottle (or baby food) simultaneously, so everyone can sit down and eat together. Two microwaves also cuts the time needed to heat leftovers in half, e.g., pizza, Chinese food, lasagna, homemade leftovers, etc. A basic Microwave can be bought for as little as $50.*

6. Save leftovers.

Given number 5, this is obvious. Leftovers can save you time. Even if you can't think of a use for a particular leftover, save it for a couple of days anyway. You can always throw it away later if you don't end up using it.

7. No special orders ever.

We try to make food that everyone likes but, alas, we don't always succeed. Nevertheless, make sure everyone in your home knows that you don't take special orders. The whole idea behind making breakfast, lunch, and dinner as efficiently as possible is that you make the same meal for everyone. If you start taking special orders, then it's going to take you a lot longer than 15 minutes to prepare and give you more to clean up. Don't!

> *Making the brood the same food means not taking special orders. If you take special orders, it's going to take you a lot longer than 15 minutes to prepare and give you more to clean up.*

8. Buy help yourself snacks.

Kids love snacks. But when baby comes along, you'll want to keep interruptions to a minimum. That means snacks that are either "help yourself," easy or both. If old enough, show your kids how to get themselves a cup of water. Keep nonperishable fruit on the counter, so they can help themselves. For more, see Chapter Three "Siblings Are Self-Reliant." The ease of these snacks is also appreciated by adults tired from tending baby.

Make breakfast, lunch, and dinner time-saving ingredients do double duty at snack time. If you've chosen items for breakfast and lunch rotation as well as dinner preparation that are quick and easy, you'll find them inherently so. In other words, most time-saving ingredients are quick and easy in and of themselves and also make great, quick snacks. For instance, pre-washed baby carrots are a time-saving ingredient for dinner that makes a quick snack. Serve them straight from the bag to your kid's bowl. Cheese and cracker packages are another quick and easy snack used in lunch rotation. Kiwi, strawberries, grapes, apple sauce cups, string cheese, pickles, and popcorn, all used for breakfast or lunch rotation also make good help yourself snacks.

> *Breakfast, lunch, and dinner "time-saving ingredients" also make quick and easy snacks.*

Chapter Eight

DUPLICATE USEFUL TOOLS AND LOCATE STRATEGICALLY

1. Set up at least two baby changing areas.

2. Set up at least two locations for frequently used tools like scissors, adhesive tape, screwdriver, and hammer.

3. Buy a second microwave.

4. Put baby wipe dispensers in car and bathrooms.

5. Keep antibacterial wipe dispensers in kitchen and bathroom for quick cleanups.

6. Put a lightweight, portable footstool in each bathroom for older siblings.

When something works well, then it's often a good idea to have more than one. There are things that we use in our daily lives for which we know this so intuitively that we expect and depend on there being more than one. Trash baskets, for instance, are expected to be in just about every room of our home. How many times have you needed to throw something away and done a 360-degree turn asking, "Where's the trash?" If there's no trash can in a room, then we buy one because it's a useful device that we frequently need.

> *Buy extra baby receiving blankets to fold in half and lay over the changing pad mattress cover. When messy, they're easier to take off and wash than the changing cover. Get them at garage sales or swap meets to save money.*

There are useful tools, however, that for some reason people traditionally buy only one of, for example, scissors, adhesive tape, hammer, microwave, screwdriver. Similarly, there are useful baby items that are typically purchased as a one-off like baby changing table or mattress, diaper ointment, diaper disposal unit, box of baby wipes. Consider duplicating these items. Buying more than one can save you and your family a lot of time and energy.

Don't limit yourself to my suggestions—identify your own useful items to duplicate. Ask yourself: *Do I find myself looking for something, finding it, then moving it to different rooms of the house?* Or, *do family members often try to use the same thing at the same time?* If the answer to either question is yes, then buy more of the item.

1. Set up at least two baby changing areas.

Traditionally, parents set up one changing table in baby's room; however, if the bedroom is upstairs and baby has a dirty diaper downstairs, then it's terribly inconvenient. Do you really want to climb stairs every time you have to change the baby? Or, consider the place you plan to bathe baby. Do you want to carry diaper, ointment, towel, and wash cloth to that location for every bath? And, if baby has a dirty diaper at bath time, do you want to carry them to their changing table first to clean them up before the bath? If not, then what do you do with the dirty diaper when they go into the bath? Wouldn't it be easier to have another changing area near the bathtub with changing pad, wipes, diapers, ointment and diaper disposal unit? You could also store your baby towels and wash clothes there, and then all you'd need to remember to bring with you at bath time is the baby.

A second changing area by baby's bath also helps make bath time safer. With diapers, wipes, ointment, towels, and wash clothes close at hand, you're not tempted to leave baby alone in the tub because you forgot something. In my home, my second changing area is in my master bedroom closet a few steps from the bath where I bathe my two-month-old daughter. Her bath time doesn't include running around looking for ointment, wipes, diaper, towel, and washcloth because they're stored next to the tub. There's also a diaper disposal unit and changing table. When it's bath time, all I have to do is bring her to the bath.

> The average baby uses six to ten diapers a day or about 2,000 to 3,000 per year. Diaper disposal unit refills cost about $7-$10 and hold approx. 140 newborn diapers or 95 large diapers. That means it can cost you as much as $300 per year for diaper disposal refills. Try adding plastic grocery bags to your changing station and diaper backpack to use for dirty diapers. They're free! Using for "wee" diapers at the changing table reduces the number of refills you'll need for your diaper disposal unit.

A second changing area can be simple without a changing table. A downstairs changing station could be simply a changing pad for use on the carpet with wipes, diapers, and ointment stored on a shelf or in a cabinet. Always select a safe location for your second changing area. As you undoubtedly know, don't leave baby's side while changing a diaper and do not use a changing mattress or pad on a shelf, bureau, or any other high surface where baby has a chance of falling.

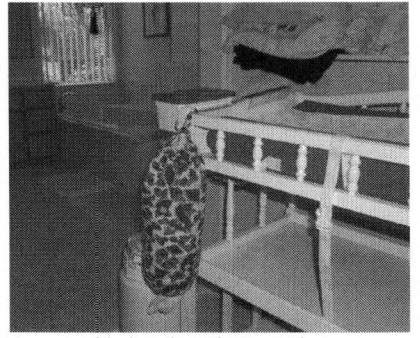

A second baby changing area in master bedroom closet within sight of bathtub.

2. Set up at least two locations for frequently used tools like scissors, adhesive tape, screwdriver, and hammer.

How many times have you found yourself looking for the scissors? You run around searching the house, and they're usually far from where you need them. And, how often have you needed adhesive tape, screwdriver, or hammer? Did you run down to the basement tool bench or out to the garage? You'll need these items

> *The laundry area is another place where scissors are useful. Store a pair in a child safe cabinet for cutting sales tags off baby clothes and other new clothes. Then they're ready to go right into the wash.*

even more often after baby arrives because, for example, you'll need a screwdriver to change batteries in baby devices that rock or vibrate and for toys. You'll also need a hammer to hang pictures of your little one. Scissors to cut tags off new baby clothes, remove irritating clothing tags, and open baby gifts. And, adhesive tape is useful generally but specifically for hanging kids' artwork and wrapping gifts for birthdays and baby showers.

Once when my mom came to visit, she opened a kitchen cabinet looking for a glass and discovered a set of tools on a shelf inside. "What's this?" she asked. "I'm sick of running to the garage for a screwdriver and hammer," I explained. The idea so impressed her that when she returned home, she set up a kitchen peg board with scissors, hammer, screwdriver, adhesive, and masking tape.

Identify sites within your home where it's helpful to have a particular tool and store it. I store a screwdriver, hammer, adhesive tape, and scissors in my kitchen because I often have kids coming there to ask me to replace batteries, wrap presents, and help with art projects. I also found myself repeatedly needing a hammer in the living room, dining room, and kitchen to hang pictures. These items are stored

> *Have packages of batteries in a variety of sizes on hand to change batteries in baby soothing devices such as bouncers and swings. Such devices may be one of the only things that quiets baby, so you don't want to run out.*

in a kitchen cabinet that my kids cannot reach.

3. Buy a second microwave.

A microwave is useful to cook meals, heat leftovers, warm baby bottles and food, pop popcorn, heat a cup of milk or hot chocolate, and so on. Therein lies a problem: microwaves are so useful that two people often want to use them at the same time.

Consider buying a second microwave. A microwave can be purchased for as little as $50. Then you can warm a baby bottle or food while you're microwaving all or part of dinner and make it possible for your family to sit down to eat a hot meal at the same time, or you can heat twice as many leftovers or cook twice as much food at once thereby cutting dinner or lunch cooking time in half.

4. Put baby wipe dispensers in car and bathrooms.

Baby wipes are good for more than just diaper changes. Keep them in your car for spills, sticky hands, faces, and replenishing diaper backpack or bag.

Additionally, baby wipes are a quick and inexpensive way to clean bathroom counters, faucets, and toilet seats. If you're toilet training, baby wipes on the bathroom counter are useful for cleaning up accidents and wiping backsides when toilet paper isn't enough.

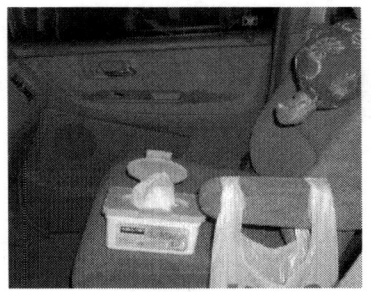

A box of baby wipes is useful in the car for spills, sticky hands or faces, and replenishing diaper backpack or bag.

5. Keep antibacterial wipe dispensers in kitchen and bathroom for quick cleanups.

Remember Chapter Seven "Fast and Frustration Free Cooking with Baby" in which I suggested that you re-evaluate your dinner recipes in light of time-saving ingredients? There's a similar time-saving revolution in the home cleaning market. The best cleaning "short cut" is antibacterial wipes. These hearty wipes contain a generous amount of antibacterial cleaner in a ready to use dispenser. They make cleaning bathrooms and kitchen faster by eliminating time-consuming steps—you no longer have to get sponge, apply cleaner to sponge, and then ring out and repeat. Just use wipe, throw out, and use the next. Wipes make quick work of cleaning counters, faucets, appliance exteriors, refrigerator shelves and doors. There are also wipes specifically for glass (mirrors and windows), stainless steel appliances, and granite or countertops.

> *When cleaning wipes run out, continue cleaning with paper towels dipped in the liquid remaining at the bottom of the container.*

6. Put a lightweight, portable footstool in every bathroom for older siblings.

Kids need footstools to brush teeth and wash hands. During toilet training days, they need stools to help them climb onto the toilet. See Chapter Three "Siblings Are Self-Reliant" for more. Make sure there's a lightweight stool in each bathroom which they can move back and forth between toilet and sink.

Chapter Nine

WHAT NEXT?

Crib Sheets takes you beyond the advice "sleep when baby sleeps." Now, you're a confident mom or dad with a plan. Your confidence comes from knowing that you've set yourself up to get the most sleep possible.

You won't waste valuable sleep time performing tasks while baby sleeps that can be done with baby awake. If a task requires more than 15 minutes of uninterrupted concentration, you'll do it with baby asleep. Since your setup to shorten such tasks in number and duration, you'll get yourself back to bed faster.

You've taught big brother and sister self-reliance, so baby and parent nap time won't be interrupted; moreover, with adults in your home also self-reliant, there's even less for you to do.

Meal time can be especially frustrating with baby, but since you've revised your meal preparation methods to fit within baby's 15-minute contentment window, meals are made quickly and stress-free.

You've also reduced the number of errands you run by car, and those you run via car you accomplish either without getting out or with getting kids in and out as quickly as possible. What next?

You're ready! But before I say goodbye, I think it's important to discuss two realities of newborn care that most parents don't truly anticipate: sleepless nights and the won't-stop-crying baby.

Chapter Ten

SLEEPLESS NIGHTS WITH BABY

Most expectant parents pay lip service to the sleepless nights ahead; however, until you're actually there night after night, it's impossible to understand how lonely and depressing it can be. The truth is your newborn will wake every two hours to feed and won't always go back to sleep. There will be many nights when you'll be up at 1, 2, or 3:00 a.m. with a fussy baby. They'll be nights where you'll be up all night long. It's lonely and frustrating. I remember spending nights pacing back and forth holding baby and whispering, "Go to sleep, little one." You feel totally alone. Your mind starts thinking all sorts of ridiculous but completely understandable thoughts like: "Why did I have a baby?" or "I'm the worst mom in the world," or "My bikini days are over," or "He gets this from his father," or "I'm never going to be able to sleep all night again," or "What if this goes on for years?"

When you're bone tired, it's difficult to think clearly. That's important to remember because it will help you take it easy on yourself. Remember that newborns are unpredictable; therefore, making them sleep is not under your control, so when you're up all night, remember it's your extreme fatigue (and perhaps hormones too) that cause you to feel lonely, frustrated, and think depressing thoughts.

These up-all-night nights are the hardest to get through. Here are some positive thoughts that helped me get through it: "At two months, he'll start to sleep longer intervals, that's not so far away," and "Millions of babies are born each year in the U.S., that means there are thousands of Moms awake right now," and "Just a few more hours and I can hand him over to dad (or grandma, or another relative)," and "It's impossible for a baby to stay awake forever; he'll fall asleep soon, and then I can too."

Sometimes it's helpful to "write off" the night. In other words, accept the fact that you're not going to get any sleep tonight. Once the night is written off, you'll feel less frustrated because your focus shifts from getting sleep to making the night fun; for example, on nights where it was clear that my bright-eyed baby wasn't going to sleep; I'd "write it off" and take them downstairs to stream a movie, or I'd bring them along to make myself a delicious snack.

    This brings me to my last but perhaps most effective suggestion: the best way to get through up-all-night nights is to give yourself something to look forward to. If it's possible, try to have someone available to whom you can hand the baby in the morning.

    I remember one weekend when my eldest son Eiche was only a few weeks old that he cried seemingly nonstop. We tried everything to soothe him. Finally, my husband and I put him in the bassinet and let him cry. We walked out to our backyard and stood there listening to him wail. I sobbed. Paul hugged me and said, "Wait here." He returned with a beer for himself and a glass of wine for me. We sat on the deck, and he said, "Are you thinking what I'm thinking?" I knew what he was thinking. "Why did we have a baby?" I said sadly. "We're the worst parents ever." Eiche continued crying. After a few minutes, Paul called his mom. He said, "Mom, listen to this..." holding the phone over Eiche, so she could hear him cry. When Paul got back on the phone, he heard her say, "That poor baby; I'm coming over!" She hung up. "We're about to get a break," he said hugging me again.

    With my second child, I had the foresight to ask a relative (great grandma) to live-in for the baby's first few weeks. We had an arrangement whereby I would have the baby all night, but great grandma would take him at 6:00 am for two hours (or longer if there was breast milk in the refrigerator). Knowing that relief was a few hours away made being up all night with a fussy baby much easier. Just that little bit of hope made all the difference in my outlook and mood. I wish I had done that with my first child.

Chapter Eleven

THE WON'T STOP CRYING BABY

Let's turn to the "won't stop crying" baby. The truth is, unfortunately, that even if you somehow end up with an angel baby, there will be times when they cry nonstop. Thankfully, for most infants these episodes are few. Make sure to check diaper, see if they want to eat, burp them, check their clothing for anything that might pinch or stick, and cuddle. If they continue crying for an hour or more, consult a pediatrician to make sure there isn't a medical problem.

Once you're satisfied that there isn't anything medically wrong, or if there is it's something you can't do much about, for instance, colic or gas, then the question is: "How do you get through it?" This is a tough one. If you read this book, then you're already performing tasks as quickly and efficiently as possible. That helps right there. But beyond that, the most important thing to remember is it's okay to take breaks when you need too. If you feel like you really just cannot take any more of the baby, and there's no one to hand them to, then it's okay to put them in their bassinet, crib, or other safe place and let them cry for twenty minutes or so. You take a break. Read a magazine or have a cup of coffee. Take a lemonade into the backyard and smell the fresh air. Watch TV. Do whatever you enjoy. After twenty minutes, go get baby and try something new.

Remember that you have options. A change of scenery may do you both good Try strollering your little one around the block or a park. How about taking them for a drive? Driving often soothes babies. Try a stroller ride through the mall. Malls are great places to take a fussy baby because they're entertaining and have things you both need—coffee, restrooms with changing tables, air conditioning, drugstore for baby supplies, places to sit down, and shops to enjoy. Also, there's always grandma and grandpa or other relatives. Call and see if they can take your baby for a while, or maybe they'd enjoy it if you and baby came over for lunch or dinner?

I hope this book helps you find more time to enjoy your new family. All the insight and advice offered herein I learned while in the trenches with my newborns. I think you'll find the sleep maximizing strategies effective and well worth it. After your little one starts sleeping four-hour intervals and then through the night, you'll find that your *Crib Sheets'* techniques continue saving time. Only now you'll be able to use your extra time for other things you enjoy besides catching up on sleep. Take care, and God bless you and your precious family.

About the Author

Attorney turned award-winning author Elizabeth Gardner has been coaching students into selective colleges like the University of Virginia, the University of North Carolina Chapel Hill, Duke University, Princeton University, Yale University, and the University of Cambridge since 2008. Her books *Coach Mom Top College Admission Playbook* and *Standing Out by Stepping Back The Zen of Getting into Selective Colleges* were published in 2021 and 2023.

A successful author in the parenting genre, her books *Crib Sheets New Parent Sleep Solutions* and *Canny Granny How to Be the Favorite Grandparent* are Mom's Choice Award® recipients. Elizabeth lives a happy, quiet life in Weaverville, North Carolina.

Made in the USA
Columbia, SC
22 March 2024